Phacoemulsification Made Easy

Phacoemulsification Made Easy

Aasheet H Desai DOMS FRCS Ophth (Edin)
Ophthalmic Surgeon, Prince Charles Eye Unit
King Edward VII Hospital, Windsor

Jack J Kanski MD MS FRCS FRCOphth
Honorary Consultant Ophthalmic Surgeon
Prince Charles Eye Unit
King Edward VII Hospital, Windsor

Commentary by Ray Willment

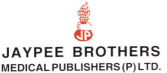

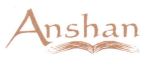

First published in the UK by

Anshan Ltd
in 2006
6 Newlands Road
Tunbridge Wells
Kent TN4 9AT, UK

Tel/Fax: +44 (0)1892 557767
E-mail: info@anshan.co.uk
www.anshan.co.uk

Copyright © 2006 by (authors)

The right of (authors) to be identified as the author of this work has been asserted in accordance with the Copyright, Designs and Patents act 1988.

ISBN 1 904798 659

British Library Cataloguing in Publication Data
A catalogue record for this book is available from the British Library

All rights reserved. No part of this publication may be reproduced, stored in a retrieval system, or transmitted in any form or by any means, electronic, mechanical, photocopying, recording and/or otherwise without the prior written permission of the publishers. This book may not be lent, resold, hired out or otherwise disposed of by way of trade in any form, binding or cover other than that in which it is published, without the prior consent of the publishers.

Printed in India by Gopsons Papers Ltd., A-14, Sector 60,Noida

Many of the designations used by manufacturers and sellers to distinguish their products are claimed as trademarks. Where those designations appear in this book and where the publisher was aware of a trademark claim, the designations have been printed in initial capital letters.

PREFACE..............................

Cataract is the most common cause of blindness worldwide. Phacoemulsification is the mainstay for cataract surgery in the developed countries and is increasing in popularity in the developing countries.

This book is aimed at the trainee ophthalmologist and succinctly illustrates the various steps in phacoemulsification. The attached CD-ROMs contains videos with instructions. The initial steps in the procedure are shown in slow motion.

AHD would like to acknowledge the input of Mr. Richard Packard in his formative years as a cataract surgeon.

Aasheet H Desai
Jack J Kanski

CONTENTS

1. Preoperative Considerations ----------------- 1
2. Anaesthesia -------------------------------------- 21
3. Preparation for Surgery ---------------------- 33
4. Phacodynamics --------------------------------- 43
5. Phacoemulsifiers ------------------------------- 49
6. Paracentesis and Incision -------------------- 55
7. Viscoelastics ------------------------------------- 67
8. Capsulorrhexis ---------------------------------- 71
9. Hydrodissection -------------------------------- 81
10. Phacoemulsification -------------------------- 89
11. Irrigation and Aspiration ------------------- 117
12. Insertion of IOL and Completion -------- 121
    Index --- *131*

VIDEO CONTENTS................

CD 1

1. Peribulbar anaesthesia
2. Sub-Tenon anaesthesia
3. Draping
4. Making sideports
5. Wound construction
6. Capsulorrhexis
7. Hydrodissection

CD 2

8. Soft cataracts
9. Grade 3 cataracts
10. Hard cataracts
11. Irrigation and aspiration
12. Inserting IOL

Chapter 1

Preoperative Considerations

OCULAR HISTORY

Trauma

Blunt Trauma

Blunt trauma may result in a fine tremor of the lens on eye movement (phacodonesis) due to zonular dehiscence (Fig. 1.1). In this situation a capsular tension ring may be required to stabilize the lens after hydrodissection. Higher settings of vacuum and power should be used to reduce the stress on the zonules.

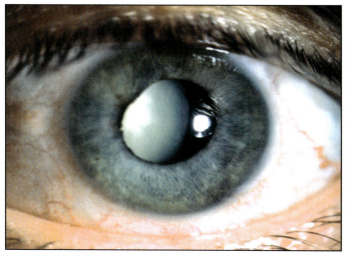

Fig. 1.1: Blunt trauma causing zonular dehiscence and lens subluxation.

Penetrating Trauma

Penetrating trauma may be associated with damage to the posterior capsule with an increased risk of a dropped nucleus during surgery.

Refraction

High Myopia

High myopia, especially when associated with a posterior staphyloma, carries an increased risk of globe perforation during peribulbar anaesthesia. A highly myopic eye may also have an unstable anterior chamber and mobile posterior capsule. The more myopic eye may also be amblyopic.

Hypermetropia

Very hypermetropic eyes may require two intraocular lens (IOLs) implants one on top of the other (piggyback).

MEDICAL HISTORY

Diabetes

Diabetic Retinopathy

Diabetic retinopathy should be treated prior to cataract surgery, if possible (Fig. 1.2). Proliferative diabetic retinopathy and macular oedema may develop or worsen following cataract surgery.

Other Problems

Other problems in diabetic patients include small pupils, pigment dispersion, delayed wound healing, fibrinous uveitis and an increased risk of infection.

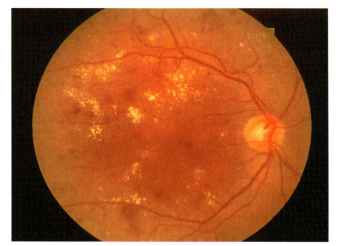

Fig. 1.2: Diabetic retinopathy should be treated prior to cataract surgery.

> *NB:* Occasionally the main purpose of cataract surgery is to improve visualization of the fundus for management of diabetic retinopathy. A large capsulorrhexis is recommended.

Other Considerations

Hypertension

Hypertension may rarely increase the risk of suprachoroidal (expulsive) haemorrhage.

Anticoagulants

Warfarin (INR should be less than 2.5) can be stopped three days prior to surgery in consultation with a haematologist. If possible, topical anaesthesia should be used to decrease the risk of bleeding.

EXAMINATION

Grading of Nucleus

One of the important factors to be considered for successful cataract surgery involves judging the hardness of the nucleus. This is particularly important for surgical training, as appropriately chosen cases reduce the risk of complications. The colour of the nucleus depends on the age of the cataract and varies from transparent–grey–yellow–amber–brown–black. The latter occupies most of the lens and is the hardest. The hardness of a mature cataract is difficult to judge because the nucleus is not visible. An important consideration is the duration of visual loss; the longer the visual loss, the harder the nucleus.

Grade 1 (Fig. 1.3)
- Soft
- Transparent
- Grey.

Example: Recent cortical or subcapsular opacity.

Grade 2
- Slightly hard
- Grey or yellowish-grey.

Example: Presenile cataract.

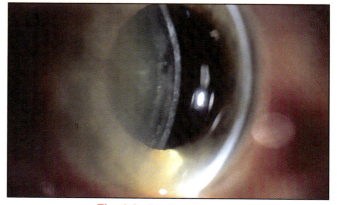

Fig. 1.3: Grade 1 nucleus.

Grade 3 (Fig. 1.4)
- Moderately hard
- Yellow with tinges of grey.

Example: Typical senile cataract.

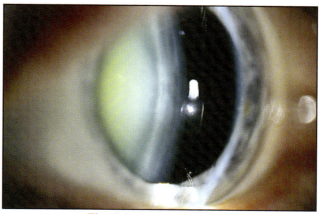

Fig. 1.4: Grade 3 nucleus.

Preoperative Considerations

Grade 4
- Hard
- Yellow-amber.

Example: Cataract in an elderly patient.

Grade 5 (Fig. 1.5)
- Very hard
- Brown or amber-black.

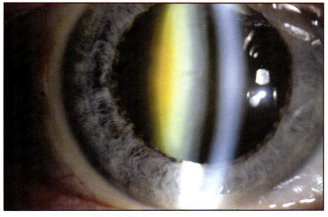

Fig. 1.5: Grade 5 nucleus.

External Features

Deep Set Eyes and Small Palpebral Fissures

Deep set eyes and small palpebral fissures are indications for a temporal incision to enhance surgical access and maneuvering of the phaco tip without being hampered by the superior orbital rim (Fig. 1.6). Annoying reflections from flooding by fluid can be eliminated by asking the patient to turn the head into the appropriate direction.

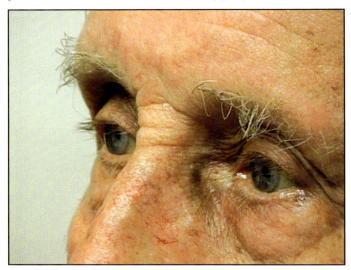

Fig. 1.6: A prominent superior orbital rim.

Hearing Aids

Hearing aids must be removed or protected from soaking during surgery (Fig. 1.7).

Staphylococcal Blepharitis

Staphylococcal blepharitis is a risk factor for postoperative endophthalmitis and must be treated prior to surgery (Fig. 1.8).

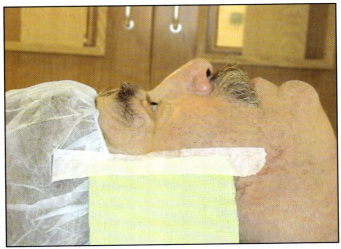

Fig. 1.7: Protection of hearing aid.

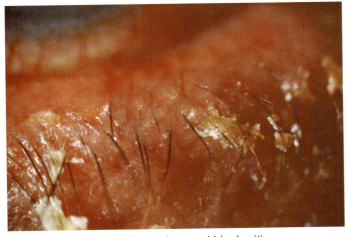

Fig. 1.8: Staphylococcal blepharitis.

Infected Contralateral Socket

Infected contralateral socket is also a risk factor for postoperative endophthalmitis (Fig. 1.9).

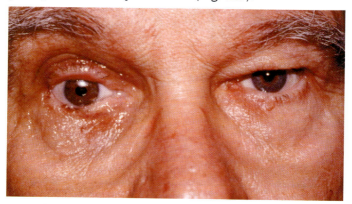

Fig. 1.9: Infected socket.

Chronic Dacryocystitis

Chronic dacryocystitis should be treated before the cataract surgery (Fig. 1.10).

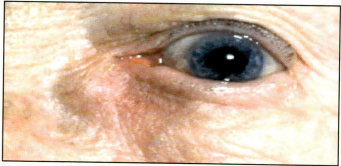

Fig. 1.10: Chronic dacryocystitis.

Cornea

Pannus and location of corneal opacities should be noted so that the incision may be planned accordingly (Fig. 1.11). A compromised endothelium (Fig. 1.12) should be protected by the judicious use of balanced salt solution plus (BSS Plus) and Viscoat.

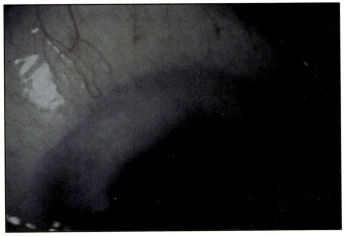

Fig. 1.11: Corneal opacities and pannus influence location of the incision.

Pupil Size

A small pupil may result in an inadequate capsulorrhexis (rhexis) with increased risk of damage to the edge of the rhexis during manipulation of the nucleus. Other problems include incomplete cortical clean-up so that small nuclear fragments may be left behind the iris because of poor visibility (Fig. 1.13). Management of a small pupil may involve one of the following:

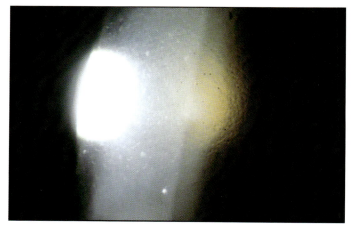

Fig. 1.12: Endothelial dystrophy should be identified before surgery.

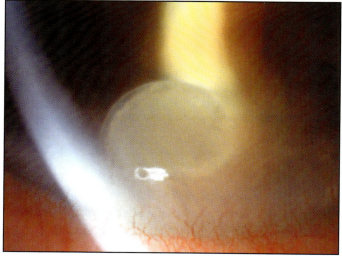

Fig. 1.13: Residual lens matter is more frequent in eyes with small pupils.

Preoperative Considerations

1. Injection of a viscoelastic between the iris and lens may break weak posterior synechiae.
2. Blunt dissection to break strong synechiae.
3. Stripping of pupillary membranes from the pupillary margin (Fig. 1.14) and stretching with forceps (Fig. 1.15).
4. Other options include use of heavy viscoelastics (Fig. 1.16) sphincterotomies, iridotomy, dilating rings or iris hooks (Fig. 1.17).

Anterior Chamber Depth

Shallow Anterior Chamber

A shallow anterior chamber is associated with overall reduction of the safe zone (Fig. 1.18). Endothelial cell loss is potentially higher from surgical trauma so that the endothelium must be protected with viscoelastics. The risk of iris trauma is increased because the angle at which the instruments are inserted is more critical than in an eye with a deeper anterior chamber (Fig. 1.19).

Very Deep Anterior Chamber

A very deep anterior chamber predisposes to trauma at the site of incision because the phaco tip must be nearly vertical when removing the nucleus. Manipulation of the nucleus may also be difficult and the increased mobility of the posterior capsule may result in capsular damage.

14 PHACOEMULSIFICATION MADE EASY

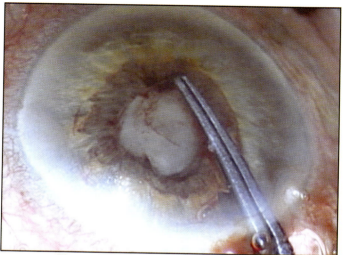

Fig. 1.14: Stripping pupillary membranes.

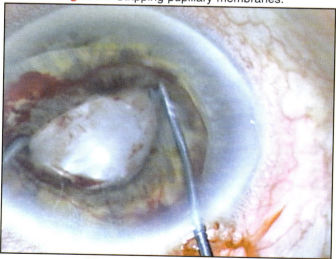

Fig. 1.15: Stretching the pupil.

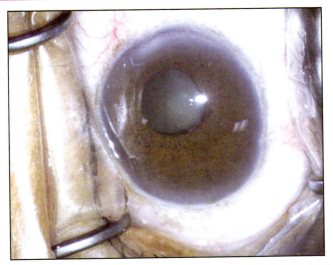
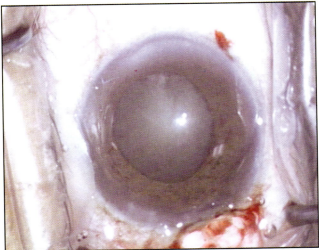

Fig. 1.16: (a) Small pupil prior to stretching (b) following stretching with heavy viscoelastics.

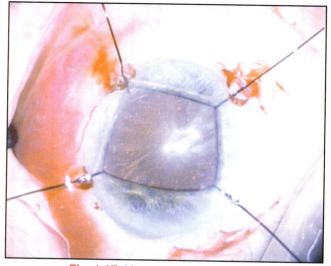

Fig. 1.17: Iris stretching with hooks.

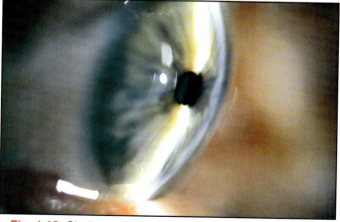

Fig. 1.18: Shallow anterior chamber decreases the central safe zone.

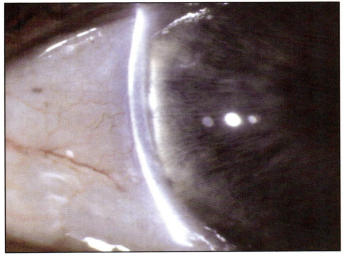

Fig. 1.19: The angle at which instruments enter the eye is more critical in an eye with a shallow anterior chamber.

ASSOCIATED OCULAR DISEASE

Uveitis

Identification of Potential Limitations

Identification of potential limitations for surgical success is important such as miosis, glaucoma band keratopathy (Fig. 1.20a), and cystoid macular oedema (Fig. 1.20b).

Control of Uveitis

Control of inflammatory activity prior to surgery is crucial to minimize complications. Ideally anterior chamber activity

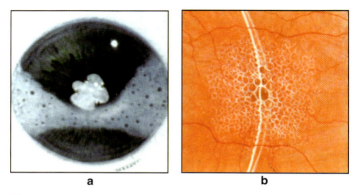

Fig. 1.20: Limitations for surgical success: (a) Band keratopathy and posterior synechiae (b) cystoid macular oedema.

should be absent or minimal (+1 cells or less) for three months prior to surgery. In quiet eyes topical steroids (prednisolone acetate 1% or dexamethasone sodium 0.1%) are used six times a day, starting one week before surgery. Patients already receiving systemic steroids should have their dose increased.

Glaucoma

Filtration Bleb

A filtration bleb should be avoided when making the incision (Fig. 1.21).

Intraocular Pressure

Intraocular pressure may rise to over 60 mm Hg during surgery so that a severely damaged optic nerve head may sustain further damage. There is also a risk of postoperative steroid-induced ocular hypertension in patients with

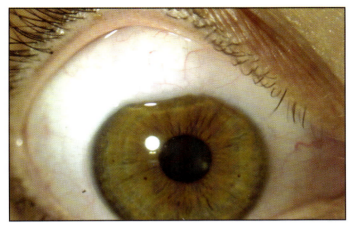

Fig. 1.21: Filtration bleb.

primary open-angle glaucoma. Prior to surgery, elevated intraocular pressure should be controlled medically. Because combined trabeculectomy and cataract surgery may result in failure of the filtering procedure it is advisable to perform glaucoma surgery six months before cataract surgery.

Previous Vitrectomy

Uncertain Visual Outcome

Visual outcome may be uncertain because of pre-existing retinal pathology.

Lack of Vitreous Support

Lack of vitreous support may result in increased stress on the zonules, an excessively mobile posterior capsule and an increased risk for capsular tear.

Other Factors

Sudden and paradoxical changes in size of pupil along with fluctuations in anterior chamber depth may put extra stress on the zonules. When the infusion is started the pupil dilates and the anterior chamber deepens; when the infusion is turned off the pupil constricts and the anterior chamber shallows.

Pseudoexfoliation

Pseudoexfoliation is associated with poor pupillary dilatation and weak zonules (Fig. 1.22). A capsular tension ring may minimize the risk of dropping the lens into the vitreous.

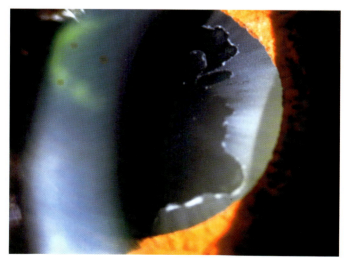

Fig. 1.22: Pseudoexfoliation is associated with weak zonules and poorly dilating pupils.

Chapter 2

Anaesthesia

Anaesthesia may be: (a) *topical*, (b) *infiltrative* or (c) *general*. Akinesia is less important but is useful during the paracentesis, wound construction and capsulorrhexis. Analgesia is adequate with drops but more complete and prolonged with sub-Tenon and peribulbar injections.

TOPICAL ANAESTHESIA

Topical anaesthesia is the preferred method as it is inexpensive and leads to faster turnover of surgery with quicker visual rehabilitation. Anaesthetic agents include lignocaine gel, proxymetacaine, benoxinate and amethocaine (Fig. 2.1). Unpreserved lignocaine 1% may be used as hydrodissection fluid.

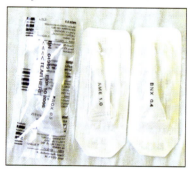
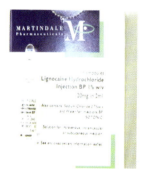

Fig. 2.1: Topical anaesthetics.

Advantages

1. The eye does not roll when moving the phaco probe because the intrinsic tone of the extraocular muscles is preserved. This is particularly useful when using the

temporal incision because the range of horizontal eye movements is larger than vertical.
2. The patient can be asked to change gaze when making side-port incisions. This applies particularly to patients with deep set eyes or smaller palpebral fissures when negotiating the bridge of the nose or superior orbital rim.
3. Subconjunctival haemorrhage does not occur.
4. The nerves controlling the eye movements and the optic nerve are not affected resulting in faster visual rehabilitation and no risk of diplopia.

Disadvantages

1. Eye movement during capsulorrhexis may result in an inappropriate tear.
2. Patients who are hard of hearing are not suitable because cooperation and communication are essential.
3. Tendency to squeeze the fellow eye will cause undue contraction of the orbicularis of the eye being operated. The patient should be asked to keep both eyes open.

NB: If applanation tonometry can be performed without a struggle, the patient will probably be suitable for topical anaesthesia.

INFILTRATIVE ANAESTHESIA

Infiltrative anaesthesia may be sub-Tenon or peribulbar. The agents (Fig. 2.2) used are as follows:

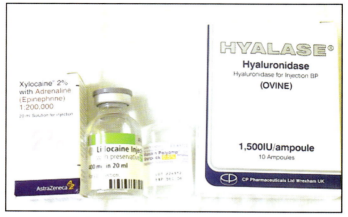

Fig. 2.2: Local anaesthetic agents and adjuncts for infiltrative anaesthesia.

1. Bupivacaine lasts in excess of 4 to 6 hours but has a slow onset.
2. Lignocaine has a very quick onset of action but this wears within about 45 minutes and is therefore usually combined with bupivacaine. Adding adrenaline also increases the duration of action and lessens the risk of bleeding. Hyalase enhances even distribution of anaesthetic around the globe.

Sub-Tenon Injection

Sub-Tenon anaesthesia is very safe because it does not involve needles which can perforate the globe. It has the added advantage of improving access in a deep set eye because it causes slight bulging of the globe as the fluid tracks in the sub-Tenon space.

Technique

1. Instill a topical anaesthetic into the conjunctival sac.
2. Insert a speculum.
3. Ask the patient to look up and out to expose the inferonasal conjunctiva.
4. Hold the forceps perpendicular to the globe, press down firmly to grasp and lift up the conjunctiva and Tenon capsule. If the forceps are not held perpendicularly, Tenon capsule will not be adequately grasped and the correct surgical plane not achieved with resultant ballooning of the conjunctiva.
5. Cut down to bare sclera with scissors (Fig. 2.3).
6. Dissect between the sclera and Tenon capsule, by inserting closed curved spring scissors along the curvature of the globe close to the sclera and then opening the scissors (Fig. 2.4).
7. Hold a syringe filled with 5 ml of anaesthetic and a sub-Tenon cannula, almost parallel to the surface of the eye.
8. Advance the cannula close to the sclera along the curvature of the globe (Fig. 2.5).
9. When the syringe has attained a near vertical orientation, inject about 3 ml (Fig. 2.6).

Problems

1. *Forward displacement of the globe:* stop injecting because further injection will increase vitreous pressure without providing any additional benefit.

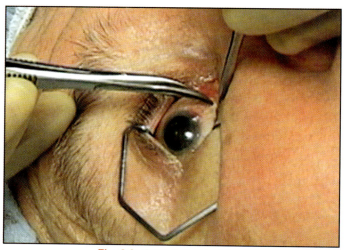

Fig. 2.3: Conjunctival incision.

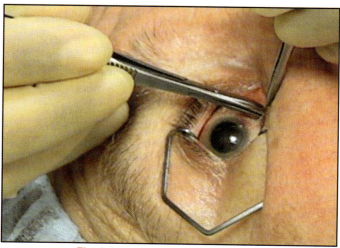

Fig. 2.4: Dissection of Tenon capsule.

ANAESTHESIA

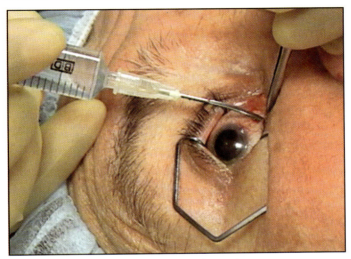

Fig. 2.5: Insertion of cannula.

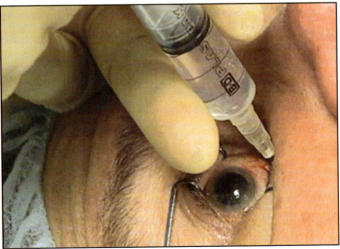

Fig. 2.6: Injection of anaesthetic.

2. *Leakage around the conjunctival edges:* push the cannula further forwards and orient the syringe more vertically.
3. *Ballooning of the conjunctiva:* stop and re-grasp the conjunctiva and Tenon more firmly and dissect down to the correct plane.

Peribulbar Injection

A peribulbar injection is made outside the cone of extraocular muscles. The diffusion of anaesthetic to the muscles will also provide akinesia.

Technique

1. Draw up the anaesthetic in a 10 ml syringe fitted with a short orange needle.
2. Ask the patient to look vertically up towards the ceiling; a cross marked on the ceiling may act as a target (Fig. 2.7).
3. With the index finger of the left hand, fixate on the inferior orbital rim and simultaneously push the globe upwards. The space thus created is used to insert the needle.
4. Push the needle through the skin into the peribulbar space (Fig. 2.8). Orientation of the needle should be at 45° to the horizontal plane, aiming towards the imagined pituitary fossa.
5. Advance about two-thirds the length of the needle.

ANAESTHESIA

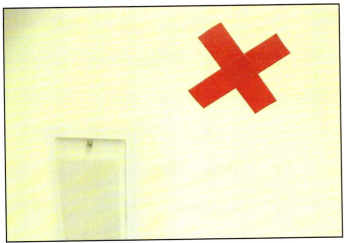

Fig. 2.7: Fixation target.

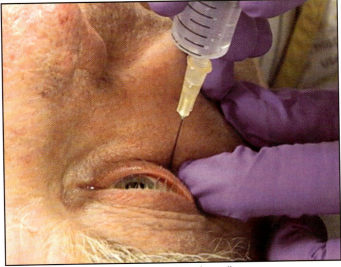

Fig. 2.8: Insertion of needle.

6. Aspirate: if blood is drawn withdraw the needle.
7. When you are confident that the needle is not inside a blood vessel inject 5-7 ml (Fig. 2.9) whilst watching for forward displacement of the globe and the drooping and fullness of the upper lid. Wrinkles on the upper lid skin usually also disappear as the anaesthetic is injected.
8. Press firmly down against the eye and massage. This enhances distribution of the anaesthetic and may also stop the spread of haemorrhage, if this has occurred.

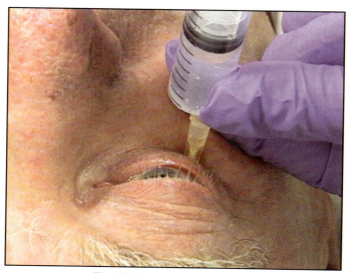

Fig. 2.9: Injection of anaesthetic.

Problems

1. *Globe perforation* is rare but special care should be taken in eyes with long axial lengths.
2. *Peribulbar haemorrhage* is usually innocuous.

GENERAL ANAESTHESIA

General anaesthesia is required in children and occasionally adults who are either extremely anxious or unable to cooperate with the surgeon's instructions.

Chapter 3

Preparation for Surgery

POSITION OF THE TABLE AND HEAD

1. The cheeks and brows should be in the same horizontal plane. This ensures that coaxial illumination provides a good red reflex and ensures easy access to the surgical field.
2. Modification of the operating table is important especially in patients who are unable to lie flat (Fig. 3.1a and b). Relatively straightforward surgery may become complicated because of incorrect positioning.

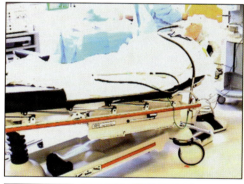

Fig. 3.1a and b: Table modification in patients unable to lie flat.

PREPARATION OF THE EYE

1. Instill topical anaesthetic into the conjunctival sac.
2. After about one minute instill 5% povidone iodine (Fig. 3.2).

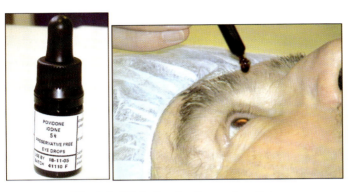

Fig. 3.2: 5% iodine for the conjunctiva.

3. Clean the skin with 10% povidone iodine (Fig. 3.3).

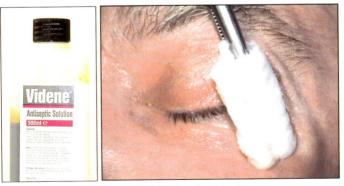

Fig. 3.3: 10% iodine for the skin.

4. Dry the skin thoroughly starting near the inner canthus and then centrally. A moist skin will impair adhesion of the drape and result in leakage of BSS into the patient's ear and hair.
5. Drape the lids and insert the speculum, making sure that the lashes are well tucked in and separated from the operating field (Fig. 3.4 and 3.5).

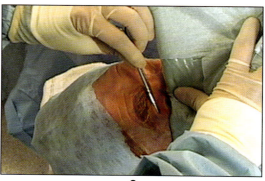

a

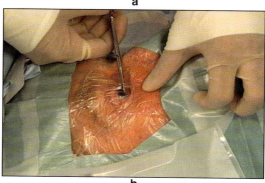

b

Fig. 3.4a and b: Draping.

PREPARATION FOR SURGERY 37

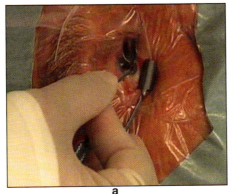

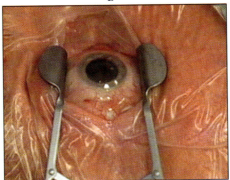

Fig. 3.5a and b: Insertion of the speculum.

MICROSCOPE SETTINGS

1. Check that the interpupillary distance is correct (Fig. 3.6).
2. Adjust the refraction on the eyepieces to your specifications (Fig. 3.7).

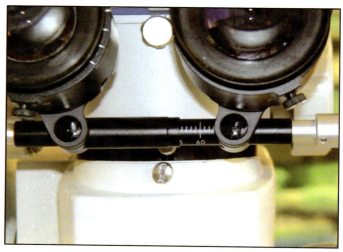

Fig. 3.6: Setting interpupillary distance.

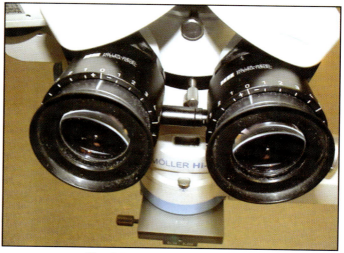

Fig. 3.7: Checking of refraction.

Preparation for Surgery

3. Center the microscope on the X, Y and Z axes by pressing the centration button.
4. Check filters and light levels. The illumination should be low when operating under topical anaesthesia. Look at the manual for the function of each individual filter (Fig. 3.8).

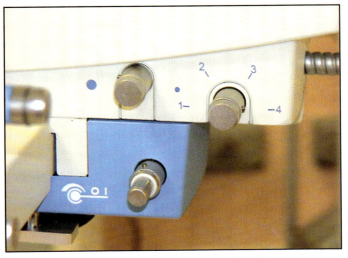

Fig. 3.8: Adjustment of filters and settings.

5. Place the microscope foot pedal within easy reach.
6. Adjust the magnification (Fig. 3.9).

NB: Too high magnification may cause loss of focus during small changes in the depth of the anterior chamber.

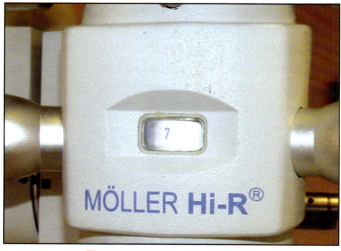

Fig. 3.9: Magnification settings.

Foot Pedal

The foot pedal is traditionally placed near the dominant foot.

Positions (Fig. 3.10)

- Position 1: The valve is opened and irrigation is gravity driven.
- Position 2: Aspiration begins and vacuum is generated if occlusion occurs—irrigation continues.
- Position 3: Phacoemulsification power begins—irrigation and aspiration continue.

There are two buttons on either side of the foot pedal which can be individually programmed. Generally a kick

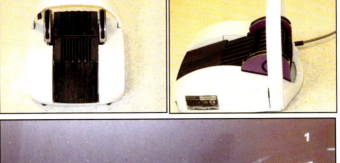

Fig. 3.10: Foot pedal and its different positions.

to the right causes reflux which may be activated if capsule is inadvertently caught in the phaco tip.

COMMUNICATION

The patient should be provided with clear instructions on how to communicate with the surgeon. This may involve squeezing a nurse's hand or operating a clicking device when wishing to communicate. This is to ensure that movement of the mouth and head does not adversely affect surgery.

Chapter 4

Phacodynamics

The importance of a clear understanding of the machine dynamics and the interaction of fluidics in tackling different forms of cataracts cannot be overstated. The various types of machines behave differently but the basic mechanism is similar. Choosing appropriate settings which are most suited to an individual's style makes surgery easier and safer (Fig. 4.1).

IRRIGATING BOTTLE

The level of the irrigation bottle is measured from the level of the patient's eye. The purpose of having the bottle at a specific height is to maintain a formed and stable eye at a reasonable intraocular pressure. The infusion flow is proportional to the height of the bottle and is dependent on gravity. In a closed system where there is no loss of fluid from the eye (neither leakage nor aspiration), the intraocular pressure is as follows (Table 4.1):

Table 4.1: Height of irrigating bottle and IOP in a closed system

Height of irrigating bottle	Intraocular pressure
15 cm	10 mm Hg
25 cm	18.4 mm Hg
50 cm	36.8 mm Hg
75 cm	55.2 mm Hg
100 cm	73.6 mm Hg
150 cm	100.4 mm Hg
200 cm	147.2 mm Hg

However, these values pertain to a closed system and factors that determine the height settings are the aspiration flow rate (AFR) and leakage around the incisions.

ASPIRATION FLOW RATE

Aspiration flow rate (AFR) refers to the volume of fluid removed from the eye. For a greater AFR the bottle must be adjusted to a higher position to compensate for increased fluid loss. In the segment removal mode, changes in AFR influence the speed of surgery, and it is recommended to tweak these settings before modifying power or vacuum. High AFR results in attraction of lens material towards the phaco tip like a magnet with faster vacuum build up and swifter removal of lens matter but with less power. However, when occlusion ceases surge increases the risk of a posterior capsular tear. The AFR should be set according to how far you would prefer to work from the capsule. If you need to go closer to the capsule use a low AFR and use high AFR if you need to work from the center of the anterior chamber.

VACUUM

The amount of negative pressure (suction) generated by the pump is indirectly controlled by the AFR (peristaltic machines). Vacuum is generated during occlusion when the pump is trying to aspirate fluid. The time taken from occlusion of the phaco tip to reach the maximum preset vacuum is called the rise time. Vacuum helps to hold nuclear material and provides the ability to manipulate lens fragments. High vacuum also decreases the need of the total power required to remove the lens.

46 PHACOEMULSIFICATION MADE EASY

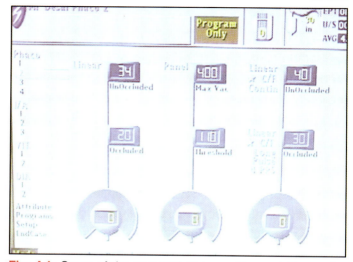

Fig. 4.1: Some of the personal phaco settings which can be altered for different types of cataract and for individual styles of operating.

SURGE

When occlusion is broken pent up energy in the system results in surge. This may cause in collapse of the anterior chamber and capsular rupture. Factors contributing to surge (Fig. 4.2) include the following:
1. Collapsible tubing.
2. High vacuum levels with high AFR. Taking the foot off the pedal and decreasing vacuum and flow when the last nuclear remnants are to be removed will decrease the risk of surge.

3. Venturi pumps cannot independently control vacuum and AFR and therefore carry a higher risk of surge.
4. Lack of provision for venting which is a mechanism for equilibrating the negative pressure in the tubing.

NB: Once the concepts of AFR and vacuum are understood they can be modified as appropriate.

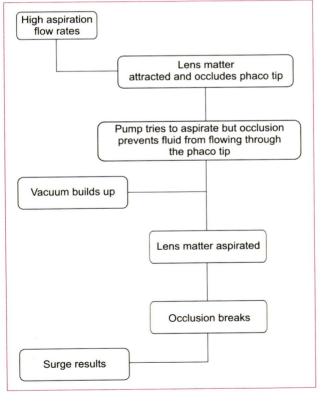

Fig. 4.2: Flow chart showing factors that contributing to surge.

Chapter 5

Phacoemulsifiers

DESIGNS

Phacoemulsifiers can be classified broadly according to how aspiration and vacuum are generated.

1. *Flow pumps* in which vacuum is indirectly controlled.
   - Peristaltic pump
   - Scroll pump
2. *Vacuum pumps* in which AFR is indirectly controlled.
   - Venturi pump
   - Diaphragmatic pump
   - Rotary vane pump

NB: Most modern machines are based on the principle of flow pumps where AFR is controlled.

HANDPIECE

The ultrasonic handpiece consists of a transducer and a titanium tip. An electronic management card supplies alternating current to the transducer which converts this to mechanical vibrations. The vibrations are expressed in terms of power by stroke length (distance covered) and frequency (number of backward and forward movement in a given time) (Fig. 5.1).

PHACO TIP

Shape

- A straight tip is most widely used.
- An angulated (Kelman) tip (Fig. 5.2a and b).

PHACOEMULSIFIERS 51

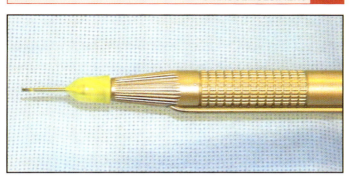

Fig. 5.1: A typical phaco handpiece with tip.

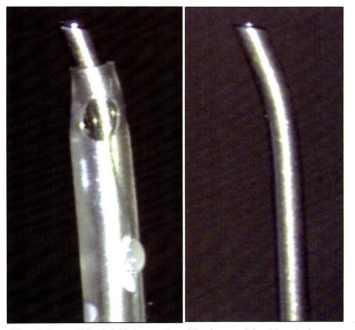

Fig. 5.2a and b: (a) Kelman tip with sleeve (b) without sleeve.

Distal Bevel

The distal bevel can be angulated through varying degrees (0°, 15°, 30° and 45°). The 45° tip will cut through a harder cataract faster because of jackhammer effect.

Diameter

- A standard tip has an outer diameter of 1.1 mm and internal diameter of 0.9 mm.
- The microtip has an external diameter of 0.9 mm and internal diameter of 0.5 to 0.7 mm. It decreases surge and is easier to occlude but requires increased vacuum settings.

Other Modifications

- A flared tip has a large diameter distal extremity.
- The aspiration bypass system (ABS) is a small hole at the edge of the phaco tip that permits continuous aspiration through the hole in the distal edge even during occlusion. This prevents surge and constantly cools the tip.

Sleeve

The sleeve protects the cornea from thermal and mechanical damage.

PHACOEMULSIFICATION

Emulsification of the lens is a result of the following phenomena:

1. *Jackhammer* pneumatic drill effect with each oscillation.
2. *Cavitation* resulting from the swift movement of solid in a liquid. At the end of each oscillation backstroke, the tip retracts and creates a vacuum which causes cavitation bubbles. The bubbles implode and release large amounts of energy causing emulsification of the lens matter (Fig. 5.3).
3. *Transmission of acoustic waves* to the tip can enhance emulsification.

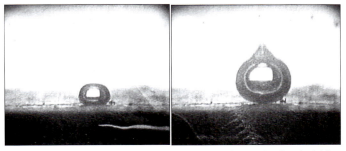

Fig. 5.3: High speed photos of formation of a cavitation bubble. (Courtesy: Dr. Larry Crum, University of Washington, Seattle).

Chapter 6

Paracentesis and Incision

The main advantage of phacoemulsification over other techniques is the ability to remove the lens through a very small incision. This obviates the need for sutures and results in faster visual rehabilitation. Three entries are made into the anterior chamber: two paracenteses and one corneal incision.

PARACENTESIS

Purposes

1. Injection of viscoelastics to maintain the anterior chamber.
2. Stabilization of the globe during surgery.
3. Manipulation of the nucleus.
4. Protection of the posterior capsule with a second instrument.
5. Irrigation and aspiration of soft lens matter.

Technique

1. Stabilization of the globe may not be necessary when operating under topical anaesthesia (Fig. 6.1). If required, it may be performed either with a 270 degree fixation ring (Fig. 6.2) or forceps for counter pressure (Fig. 6.3).
2. If using bimanual irrigation/ aspiration (I/A), the incision should be half as wide (Fig. 6.4a).
3. If using a Simcoe cannula, the incision is made with a 15-degree blade which has the same width (Fig. 6.4b).
4. The two paracenteses should be 180 degrees apart; one about 30 to 60 degrees to the left of the main

Paracentesis and Incision

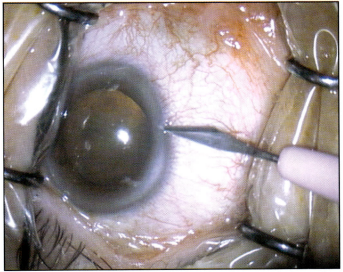

Fig. 6.1: Under topical anaesthesia muscle tone obviates the need for stabilization of the globe.

incision. The second paracentesis should be 180 degrees from the first.

Advantages of Two Sideports

1. Good anterior chamber stability with few capsular folds and less risk of a tear.
2. A formed capsular bag makes it easier to grasp cortical lens matter.
3. Less risk of iris touch.
4. Ability to crush the epinucleus and small nuclear fragments between the two instruments.
5. Safe and easy capsular polishing.

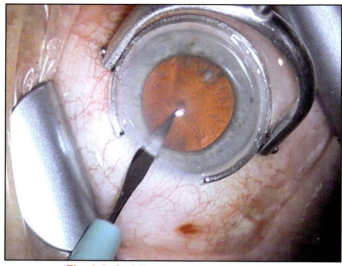

Fig. 6.2: Stabilization with a ring fixator.

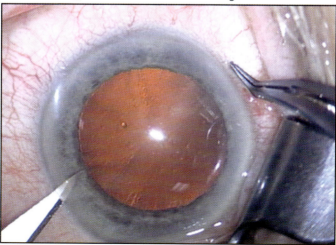

Fig. 6.3: Stabilization by counter pressure.

PARACENTESIS AND INCISION

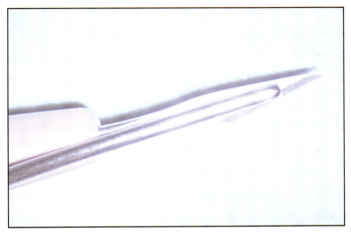

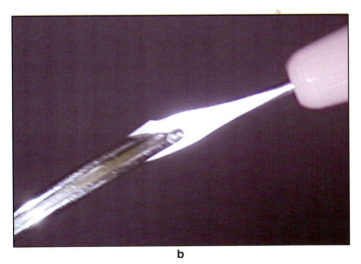

Fig. 6.4a and b: (a) Cannula used for bimanual infusion-aspiration (b) Width of Simcoe cannula compared with that of a 15 degree blade.

INCISION

Location

Clear Corneal Incision

Clear corneal incision is quick and easy but may be associated with induced astigmatism.

Limbal Incision

Limbal incision is approximately 2.5 to 3.2 mm wide and about 0.5 mm behind the edge of the vascular arcades (Fig. 6.5). It causes less induced astigmatism than a clear corneal incision but may be associated with ballooning of conjunctiva (Fig. 6.6) and bleeding into the anterior chamber when the incision is enlarged prior to IOL insertion (Fig. 6.7).

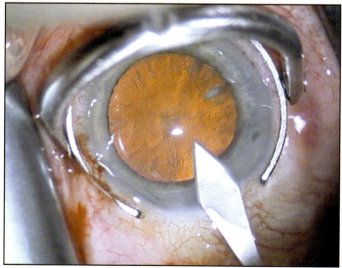

Fig. 6.5: Limbal incision.

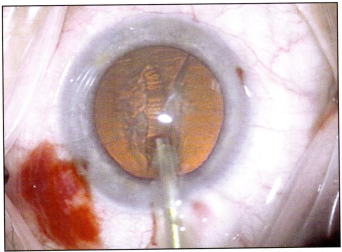

Fig. 6.6: Limbal incision associated with conjunctival ballooning.

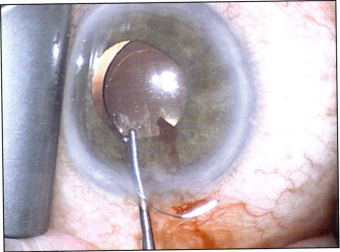

Fig. 6.7: Blood entering the anterior chamber on IOL insertion.

Sclerocorneal Incision

Sclerocorneal incision is useful if foldable IOLs are not available but has the following disadvantages:
- It cannot be performed under topical anaesthesia.
- Longer time and greater precision are required to ensure that the internal opening is corneal.
- Bleeding.
- Instrument manipulation is difficult and iris prolapse may occur.

Temporal Incision

Temporal incision is preferred for topical anaesthesia.

Advantages
- The superior orbital rim does not hinder surgery in deeply set eyes.
- Bell's phenomenon does not pose a problem.
- Less induced astigmatism because the horizontal diameter of the cornea is widest.
- A glaucoma filtration bleb or future trabeculectomy are not compromised.

Disadvantages
- Tendency for the eye to 'roll' nasally by the phacoemulsifier, especially if good akinesia is achieved.
- Tendency for the patient to turn the head away from the surgeon.
- Pooling of irrigation fluid nasally may cause annoying reflections.

Superior Incision

Advantages
- The surgeon's hand can rest on the patients' forehead.
- The incision is underneath the upper lid and causes less discomfort.

Disadvantages
- In deeply set eyes, the superior orbital ridge impairs access to the surgical field.
- In eyes with small palpebral fissures, Bell's phenomenon interferes with insertion and manipulation of instruments.

Superotemporal Incision

Superotemporal incision is a compromise between a superior and a temporal incision.

On-axis Phaco Incision

On-axis phaco incision is placed on the steeper axis according to keratometric reading; astigmatism of up to 1 D can be neutralized.

Shape

1. A single-plane stab.
2. Two-plane.
3. A three-plane incision which should have a thin posterior lip to enhance its self-sealing valve-like properties.

Technique of a Three-Plane Incision

1. Make a vertical stab in the cornea with the keratome (Fig. 6.8a).

2. Rotate the keratome horizontally and advance in the corneal plane to make a 1.5 to 2 mm long tunnel (Fig. 6.8b and c).

> *NB:* A shorter tunnel may not be self-sealing, and a longer tunnel may induce corneal folds.

3. Rotate the keratome vertically and gently advance until it enters the anterior chamber (Fig. 6.8d).

Figure 6.9 is a schematic diagram of a three-plane incision.

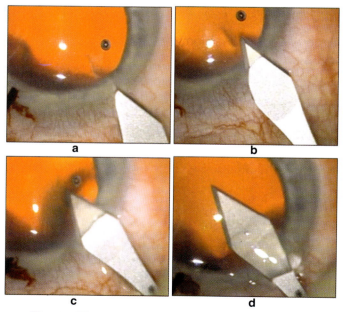

Fig. 6.8: Three plane self-sealing incision (see text).

PARACENTESIS AND INCISION 65

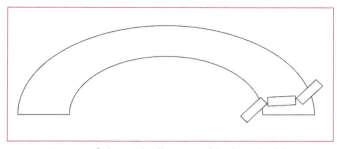

Fig. 6.9: Schematic diagram of 3 plane incision.

Chapter 7

Viscoelastics

DEFINITIONS

1. *Viscoelastics* are sophisticated biopolymers whose main constituents are glycansaminoglycans and hydroxypropylmethylcellulose.
2. *Viscosity* is the resistance to flow, a physical property of a substance that depends on the friction of its component molecules as they slide past one another. Viscosity depends on molecular weight, concentration and temperature.
3. *Pseudoplasticity.* High pseudoplastic viscoelastics have a greater tendency to flow and therefore requires a smaller-bore cannula for injecting.
4. *Elasticity* is resistance to deformation. Long chain viscoelastics are more elastic and help to absorb deforming forces during surgery.
5. *Surface adhesion (coatability)* is the ability to adhere to surfaces including instruments and IOLs.
6. *Cohesivity* is the extent to which a viscoelastic adheres to itself.

PROPERTIES

1. *Cohesive viscoelastic (Healon, Healon 5, Healon GV and Provisc)*
   - Long chains and high molecular weight
   - Used to create and maintain intraocular spaces
   - Cause elevation intraocular pressure unless removed
   - Easy to remove.

2. *Dispersive viscoelastics (Viscoat)*
   - Low molecular weight and a tendency to break up
   - Used to coat and protect the endothelium
   - Used to create and maintain space, forming compartments
   - Do not cause elevation of intraocular pressure
   - More difficult to remove than cohesive viscoelastics.

CLINICAL USES

1. *Improving visibility* by applying a dispersive viscoelastic to the cornea.
2. *Soft shell technique* involves the injection of a dispersive and then a cohesive viscoelastic underneath. The former adheres to and protects the endothelium (Fig. 7.1).
3. *If capsulorrhexis is running out to the periphery*, injecting a high molecular weight cohesive viscoelastic will help flatten the anterior capsule, lessen the risk of the capsule running out and will push the iris away (Fig. 7.2).
4. *In small pupils* a high molecular weight viscoelastic will push the iris away from the lens and induce mydriasis (see Fig. 1.16).
5. *In small posterior capsular tears* a dispersive viscoelastic (Viscoat) will push the vitreous back into the posterior chamber and plug the capsular defect.

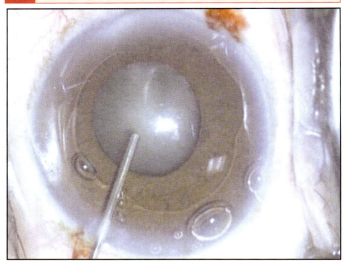

Fig. 7.1: Soft shell: Healon being injected underneath Viscoat.

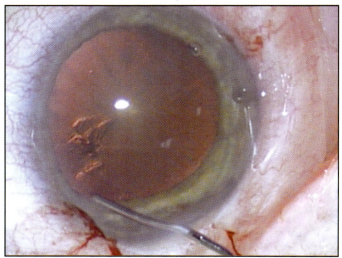

Fig. 7.2: Viscoelastic pushing away the iris and flattening the capsule.

Chapter 8

Capsulorrhexis

PRINCIPLES

A continuous central curvilinear capsulorrhexis is a very important step in phacoemulsification for the following reasons:

1. It ensures safe endocapsular surgery and hydro-dissection because the rhexis is strong and resistant to stretching.
2. It permits insertion of a posterior chamber IOL, even in the event of posterior capsular tear and vitreous loss.
3. Cortical removal of lens matter is quick and safe as there are no flaps.
4. It helps centralize the IOL.
5. Virtual elimination of uveitis–glaucoma–hyphema (UGH) syndrome and pigment dispersion.

NB: An incomplete or broken rhexis can be disastrous because it may extend across and around the lens resulting in its dislocation into the vitreous.

TECHNIQUE

Capsulorrhexis involves two movements: (a) *shearing* in which a tangential vector force is applied along the direction of the tear (Fig. 8.1) and (b) *ripping* in which a centripetal vector force strains and tears the capsule (Fig. 8.2). Ideally, the rhexis should be 0.5 to 1 mm smaller than the diameter of the optic of the IOL (i.e. approx 5 to 6 mm in diameter). It is performed as follows:

CAPSULORRHEXIS

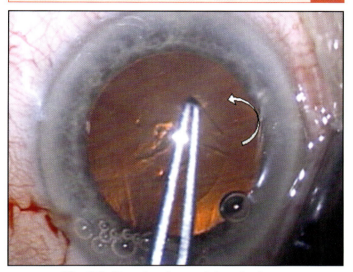

Fig. 8.1: Shearing: tangential vector force.

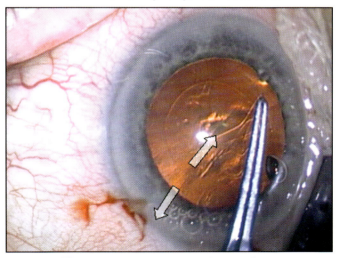

Fig. 8.2: Ripping: centripetal vector force.

1. Fill the anterior chamber with viscoelastic.
2. With a cystitome or bent needle make the initial cut in the capsule. Start from the center, pierce the capsule and move radially, cutting linearly across and fold the capsule over itself (Fig. 8.3 and 8.4).

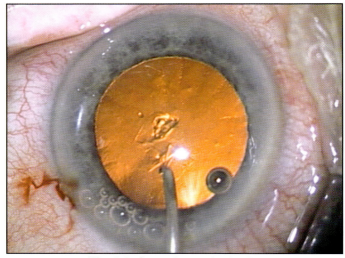

Fig. 8.3: Start of capsulorrhexis.

3. Lift up the capsule to minimize distributing the cortex and enhance visualization of the flap (Fig. 8.5).
4. With the capsule lifted, direct the forceps along the inside the curve of pupillary margin; the tangential vector force will result in a controlled circular tear (Fig. 8.1).
5. Pull centripetally to maintain a circular edge.

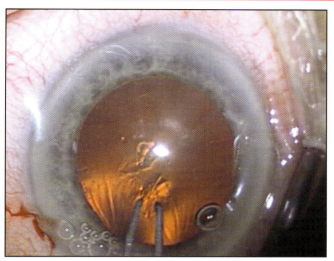

Fig. 8.4: Capsule flap folded over itself.

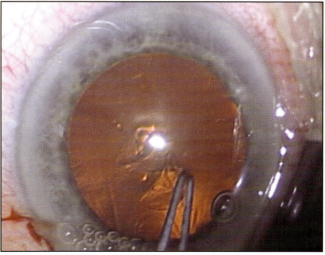

Fig. 8.5: Lifting up of capsular flap.

6. Re-grip frequently because gripping close to the edge of the tear will result in a smooth and controlled tear.
7. Bring the excess capsule to the center and then release (Fig. 8.6). This provides a clear radial edge and a flap that is easy to re-grasp.
8. Avoid exerting pressure on the posterior lip of the incision as this may result in loss of viscoelastic and 'running out' of the rhexis.
9. When completing the rhexis try to overlap it with the initial cut.

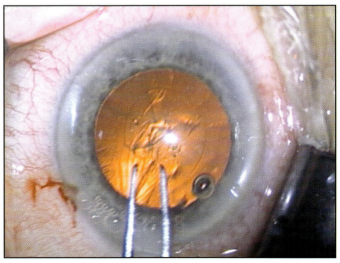

Fig. 8.6: Bring the excess capsule to the center and release.

SPECIAL SITUATIONS

Difficult Visualization of the Anterior Capsule

Difficult visualization of the anterior capsule can be remedied by injecting trypan blue (a vital dye) under air, into aqueous or under a viscoelastic. (If injecting under a viscoelastic, balanced salt solution must be injected to create a lake for the dye to stain the capsule and also prevent it coming into contact with the endothelium) (Fig. 8.7).

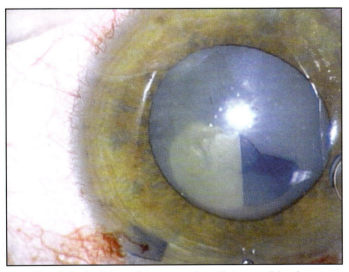

Fig. 8.7: Staining of the capsule with trypan blue in a mature cataract.

Weak Zonules

A shearing force produces less stress on zonules than a rip. It is important to use adequate Viscoat to plug the area of zonular weakness and prevent vitreous prolapse (Fig. 8.8).

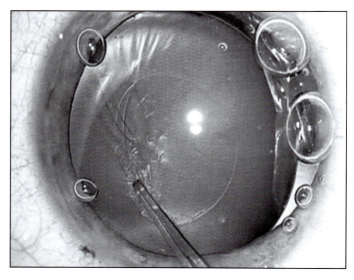

Fig. 8.8: Stress lines indicating zonular weakness.

Rhexis Running Out

This is managed as follows:
a. Stop and assess the situation.
b. Inject viscoelastic, preferably heavy Healon (GV or 5), to flatten the anterior surface of the lens and decrease

the tendency for the capsule to run out. This will also push the iris further outwards and improves visibility.
c. Hold the capsule close to the edge of the tear.
d. Pull centripetally to encourage the vector forces to tear the edge of the rhexis more centrally, away from the zonules.

NB: If resistance is encountered, the edge of the rhexis has reached the zonules and any further manipulation is dangerous. Consider converting to an extracapsular procedure or continue the rhexis from the other half and join it up to the part which has extended outwards.

Chapter 9

Hydrodissection

PURPOSE

The purpose of hydrodissection is to separate the nucleus and cortex from the capsule so that the nucleus can be more easily and safely rotated.

TECHNIQUE

1. Use a 26-gauge blunt cannula with the distal end flattened so that it appears rectangular in cross-section.
2. Make sure that the cannula is patent and attached firmly to the syringe.
3. Press gently on the posterior lip of the incision and allow some viscoelastic to egress from the anterior chamber; this is especially important if using thick viscoelastics such as Healon GV or Healon 5.
4. Insert the cannula just beneath the edge of the rhexis between 3 and 5 o'clock hours of the incision (Fig. 9.1).
5. Move the cannula gently from side to side to free the capsule from underlying cortex.
6. Tent the capsule slightly and inject fluid under the capsule. The hydrodissection wave should be easily seen provided there is a good red reflex (Fig. 9.2). When the fluid goes across the lens it will bulge forward and the anterior chamber will shallow. Too vigorous hydrodissection may result in rupture of the posterior capsule manifest as a sudden contraction of the iris.
7. As the lens prolapses forwards push it back against the posterior capsule to enable fluid trapped behind to flow anteriorly. Cleavage of cortex from the capsule

HYDRODISSECTION

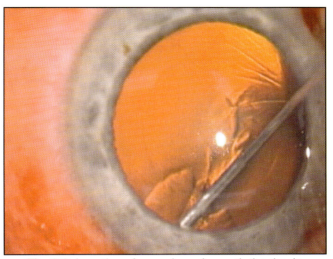

Fig. 9.1: Insertion of cannula underneath the rhexis.

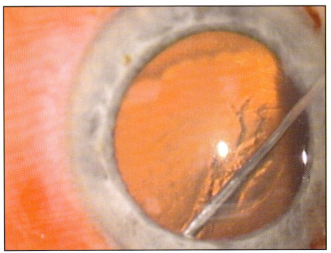

Fig. 9.2: Hydrodissection fluid wave.

will thus be completed, facilitating rotation of the nucleus (Fig. 9.3).

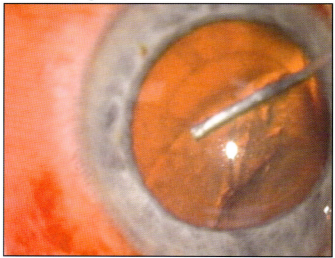

Fig. 9.3: Downward pressure on the lens to complete cortical cleaving.

8. To rotate the nucleus, place the cannula close to the edge of the rhexis, about 4 o'clock hours from the incision, and press down firmly, rotate the nucleus clockwise and then anticlockwise to reduce the stress on the zonules.

PROBLEMS

1. *Inadequate hydrodissection* will result in incomplete rotation of the nucleus with resultant strain on the

zonules. In this situation try to hydrodissect at several points to ensure cortical cleavage (Fig. 9.4).

2. *Too vigorous hydrodissection* may result in rupture of the posterior capsule (Fig. 9.5). It should be suspected if there is sudden miosis and difficulty in rotating the nucleus (Fig. 9.6 and 9.7).

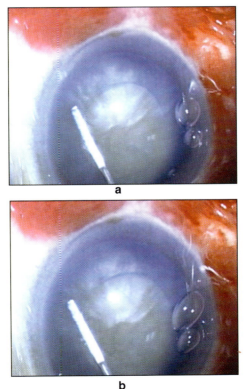

Fig. 9.4: Hydrodissection in a dense cataract. Note the subtle indentation on either side of capsular edge (b) compared to (a).

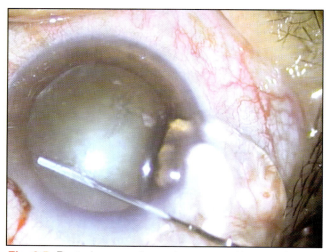

Fig. 9.5: Posterior capsular rupture caused by too vigorous hydrodissection: note egress of viscoelastic.

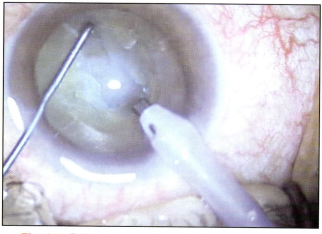

Fig. 9.6: Difficulty in rotating is indicative of posterior capsular rupture.

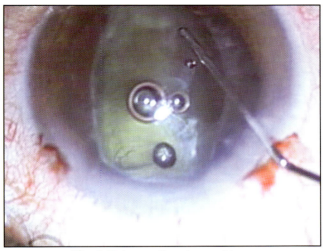

Fig. 9.7: Impending dropped lens.

Chapter 10

Phacoemulsification

The aim phacoemulsification is to remove the lens (diameter 9 mm) through a small incision without damaging adjacent structures. The technique and the machine parameters vary according to the density of the nucleus.

GRADE 3 NUCLEUS

Cataracts with grade 3 nuclei are ideal for the inexperienced surgeon because they are associated with a good red reflex, an epinuclear cushion that protects the posterior capsule, and a nucleus that is relatively easy to crack using the *'divide and conquer'* technique.

Sculpting (Divide)

Technique

1. Ensure that the microscope is central, the foot pedal correctly positioned and the phaco functional.
2. The irrigation holes on the phaco sleeves should be on either side of the bevel of the tip so that the jet of BSS squirts laterally, away from the corneal endothelium. The distal part of the tip should be left bare (Fig. 10.1) so as to provide deep narrow grooves that facilitate cracking of the nucleus; an overlong bare tip may result in a corneal burn.
3. Irrigate the cornea to remove grease and to confirm that the machine is functional (Fig. 10.2).

PHACOEMULSIFICATION

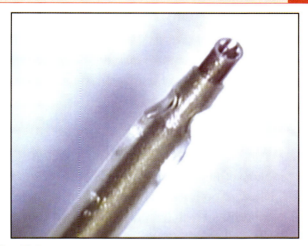

Fig. 10.1: Phaco with irrigation on either side and adequate show of the distal bare tip.

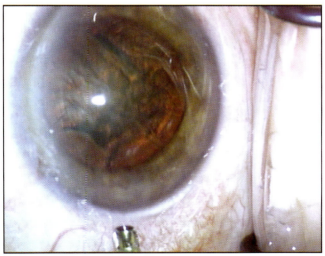

Fig. 10.2: Irrigation of the cornea.

4. Hold the incision with a notched forceps, insert the phaco tip into the eye either bevel up or bevel down (Fig. 10.3). In small pupils and shallow anterior chambers the risk of damaging the iris is less with bevel down.
5. Point the bevel upwards and aspirate superficial cortex and epinucleus (Fig. 10.4).
6. Make a long and deep trench (Fig. 10.5). The motion of the handpiece should resemble a boat, shallow at both ends and deep in the middle. The power should be highest when the tip is central and decreased as you approach the periphery.

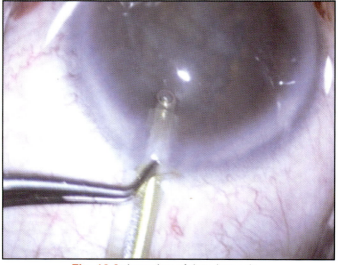

Fig. 10.3: Insertion of the phaco tip.

PHACOEMULSIFICATION

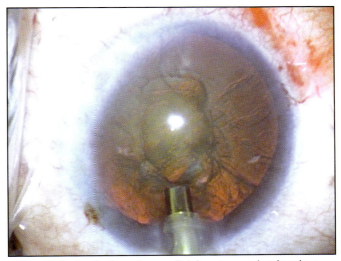

Fig. 10.4: Aspiration of superficial cortex and epinucleus.

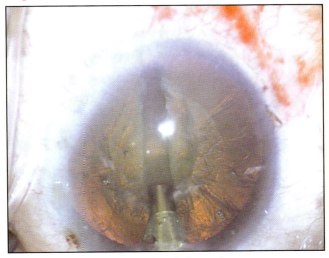

Fig. 10.5: Trench formation.

7. If the lens is excessively mobile, increase the power. If the sleeve is being caught in the borders of the trench, make the trench slightly wider.
8. The end point is reached after several passes when there is either a change in colour or the depth of the trench is twice the diameter of the tip.
9. Rotate the nucleus 180 degrees and complete the long and deep trench to make it symmetrical.
10. Rotate the lens through 90 degrees and sculpt perpendicular to the original groove.
11. Start by making a shallow groove on the proximal heminucleus. This allows greater leverage to reach at the distal heminucleus for deeper grooving.
12. Rotate 180 degrees and complete the trench (Fig. 10.6).
13. Divide the nucleus by placing the tip and the second instrument deep in the groove and then gently separate the two instruments (Fig. 10.7 and 10.8). An alternative method is to perform a crossing action to obtain better leverage for cracking.

NB: Do not press down with the instruments. The principle is akin to a "see-saw", the proximal end needs to be higher for the distal end to reach lower.

Problems

1. *Anterior chamber shallowing* may occur if the foot pedal is not maintained in position 1: continuous irrigation may be required.

PHACOEMULSIFICATION 95

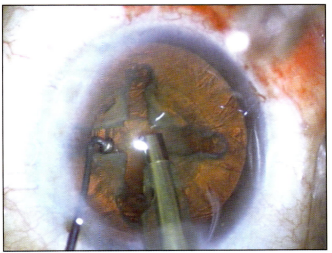

Fig. 10.6: Completion of trench formation.

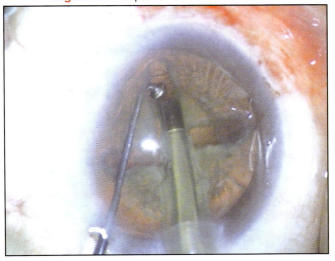

Fig. 10.7: Initial cracking of the nucleus.

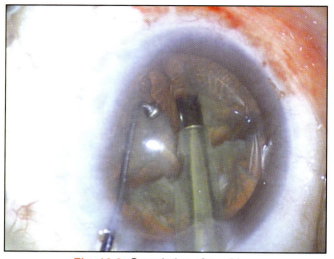

Fig. 10.8: Completion of cracking.

2. *Corneal distortion* may be caused by excessive pressure on the corneal section.
3. *Zonular weakness* is manifest by movement of the whole lens; increase the power as appropriate or use a capsular tension ring.
4. *Difficulty in cracking the nucleus*: sculpt deeper.
5. *Difficulty in rotating the nucleus* may be caused by either inadequate hydrodissection, that requires repetition, or by the presence of vitreous secondary to a posterior capsular defect.
6. *Bowl formation* may occur during cracking the shoulders of the quadrants, especially if the grooves are shallow and wide. This phenomenon may be

prevented by making the groove deep and narrow and placing the tip deep into the groove when cracking.
7. *Iris trauma* may occur when instruments enter or exit the eye; remove the manipulator before the phaco tip and ensure that the foot pedal should be in position 1 when the phaco tip is being removed (Fig. 10.9).

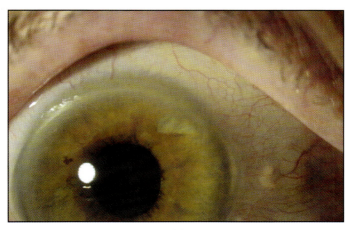

Fig. 10.9: Iris trauma.

Removal of Lens Quadrants (Conquer)

Technique

1. Using high AFR, high vacuum and low power settings. Place the tip adjacent to a quadrant and press the foot pedal to position 3.
2. Impale a quadrant with the tip by using small burst of energy (Fig. 10.10).

98 PHACOEMULSIFICATION MADE EASY

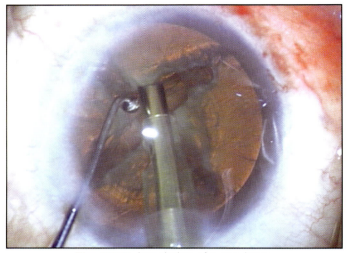

Fig. 10.10: Impalation of a quadrant.

3. Release the foot pedal to position 2 so that the tip is occluded and the machine beeps; there is maximal vacuum but no power.
4. Pull the quadrant towards the center of the anterior chamber (Fig. 10.11).
5. Steady the hand holding the phaco and resist any temptation to move the phaco tip. Use only the second instrument or the foot pedal to manipulate the nucleus once it is brought to the center.
6. Gradually increase the energy to an appropriate level dependent on the density of the lens fragment; excessive power will repel the nuclear material.

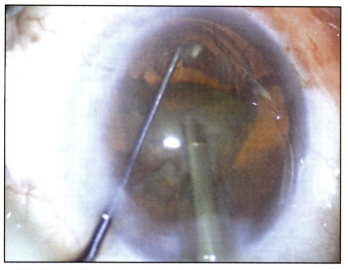

Fig. 10.11: Pulling quadrant centrally (note the epinuclear cushion behind the nucleus).

7. Repeatedly change the foot pedal position from 1 (irrigation) to 3 (power) to ensure that a fresh edge of the nuclear material presents to the tip.
8. When removing the last quadrant there is a danger of posterior capsular damage; reduce the flow and vacuum or protect the capsule by position the second instrument behind the tip (Fig. 10.12).
9. When removing the instruments from the eye the second instrument should be removed before the phaco. Avoid catching the edge of the rhexis and the iris while removing the fragments (Fig. 10.13).
10. Small nuclear fragments caught near the sideport must be removed (Fig. 10.14).

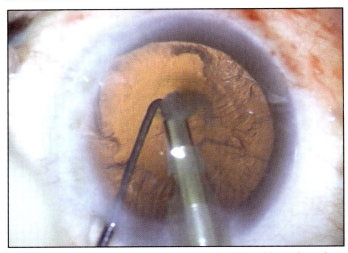

Fig. 10.12: Protection of the capsule with a blunt-tipped second instrument.

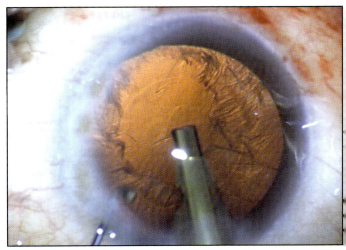

Fig. 10.13: The capsulorrhexis and iris should be avoided when removing the second instrument.

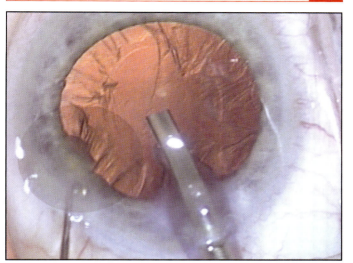

Fig. 10.14: Hidden nuclear fragments near the sideports.

Problems

1. *Inadequate separation of the nucleus* may occur, particularly when removing the first quadrant. Separation can be completed by placing the phaco tip and second instruments deeper into the groove. High AFR and vacuum settings are used to attract and pull the nucleus towards the center.
2. *Posterior capsular tear* is manifest by deepening of the anterior chamber, resistance to aspiration or emulsification as the vitreous enters the anterior chamber and plugs the phaco tip.
3. *Anterior capsular tear* may occur when sharp ended vertical choppers are used, although the anterior

capsule is sufficiently robust to sustain significant deforming forces.

4. *Endothelial trauma* may occur due to excessive ultrasonic energy and nuclear manipulation in the anterior chamber. This can be prevented by keeping the nucleus below the plane of the iris, and using a 'soft shell' technique to coat the endothelium with a dispersive viscoelastic, as previously described.

SOFT NUCLEUS

Technique

1. Make a large capsulorrhexis for better access to soft cortical material.
2. Perform meticulous hydrodissection because a soft nucleus is difficult to rotate.
3. Rotate the nucleus by going to the very edge of the rhexis to increase torque and press down firmly for easier rotation (Fig. 10.15).
4. Make very long, deep and narrow grooves to facilitate cracking. A narrow 0.9 mm gauge tip is preferred to a 1.1 mm.
5. Use very low AFR, vacuum and power so that working close to the capsule is safer.
6. Once the long grooves are formed, split the lens into two. Divide and conquer is difficult because the weak shoulders may easily break on attempted separation and result in a 'bowl formation' (Fig. 10.16 to 10.18).

PHACOEMULSIFICATION 103

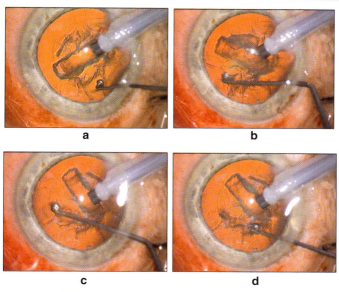

Fig. 10.15a to d: Rotation of the nucleus.

7. Remove the segments using high AFR and low vacuum. The former will attract the lens material to the tip and draw it towards the central safe zone.
8. Slice soft hemi-fragment with the blunt manipulator.

NB: There is minimal need for power as the lens is soft and pliable making it easy to aspirate with moderate levels of vacuum.

Problems

'Bowl formation' and epinuclear removal may constitute a challenge. The undivided inferior part of the lens is

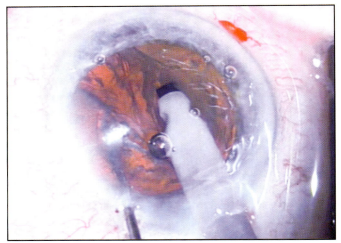

Fig. 10.16: Difficulty in separating the deeper parts of the epinucleus.

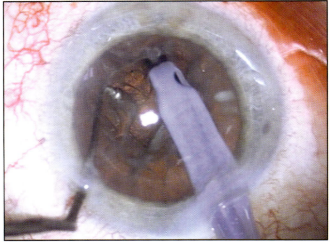

Fig. 10.17: Softer cataracts are harder to crack; the lower plates are not separated.

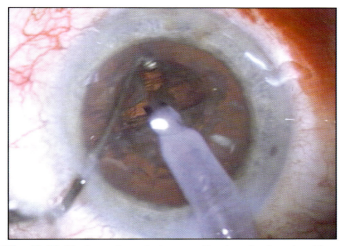

Fig. 10.18: Further attempted separation breaks the shoulders rather than cracking.

difficult to remove whilst working in close proximity to the posterior capsule (Fig. 10.19). The following steps should be taken to facilitate the procedure:

1. Use moderate flow to prevent the capsule from being attracted to the tip; very high flow may attract the capsule along with the epinucleus.
2. Use moderate vacuum. Very high vacuum is not desirable because it may result in surge and damage to the posterior capsule. Low vacuum is also inappropriate because it precludes adequate holding of lens material.
3. Inject viscoelastic underneath the capsule as in hydrodissection to provide an edge of epinuclear material and also to protect the posterior capsule.

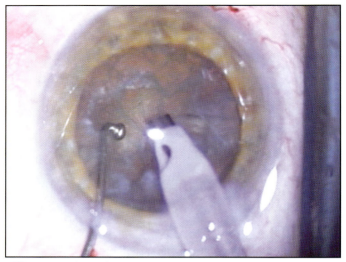

Fig. 10.19: Bowl formation; appropriate settings for flow and vacuum are necessary to work closer to the capsule.

4. Use a push pull technique as follows (Fig. 10.20):
    a. Place the manipulator in the central part of the bowl.
    b. Push the epinucleus from the center to the 6 o'clock position.
    c. Simultaneously using aspiration and vacuum pull the nucleus from underneath the capsule to the center.

HARD NUCLEUS

Technique

1. Make the corneal incision slightly wider so that the resultant leakage prevents a wound burn.

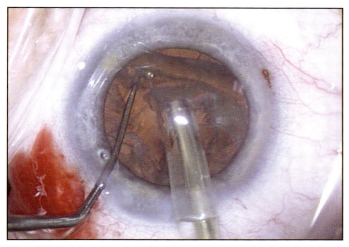

Fig. 10.20: Using a push pull technique to remove the epinucleus.

2. Inject Viscoat towards the endothelium (soft shell technique) (Fig. 10.21).
3. Make a large capsulorrhexis to facilitate access for horizontal chopping and prevent damage to the rhexis during vertical chopping (Fig. 10.22).
4. Perform hydrodissection gently because the wave is not visible. Use small amounts of fluid in multiple locations. Clues to adequate hydrodissection include forward bulging forward of the lens and the egress of viscoelastic from the eye (Fig. 10.23).
5. Rotate the lens.
6. Use phaco settings for segment removal mode with high vacuum, high AFR and moderate power.

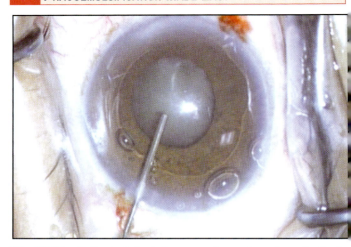

Fig. 10.21: Soft shell technique: a dispersive viscoelastic is injected towards the endothelium and a cohesive viscoelastic towards the lens.

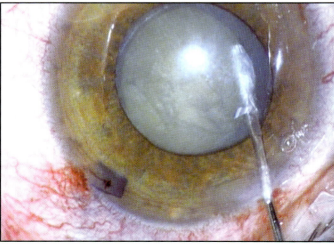

Fig. 10.22: A large capsulorrhexis is helpful in hard cataracts.

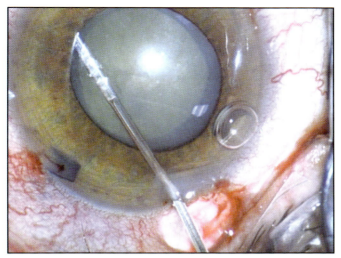

Fig. 10.23: Adequate hydrodissection: bulging forwards of the lens and egress of viscoelastic.

7. Use a chopping technique because less overall power will be required to remove lens material and there is also minimal stress exerted on the zonules.
    a. In horizontal chopping the chopper has a blunt tip and is placed horizontally underneath the capsule and then turned vertically as the equator is reached (Fig. 10.24).
    b. In vertical chopping the chopper has a pointed tip and need not be advanced beyond the edge of the capsulorrhexis (Fig. 10.25).

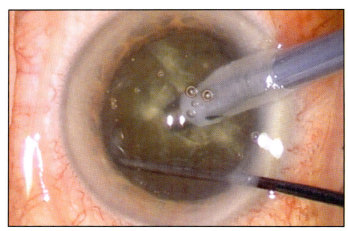

Fig. 10.24: Horizontal chopping: a blunt-tipped chopper is passed beyond the capsulorrhexis upto the equator.

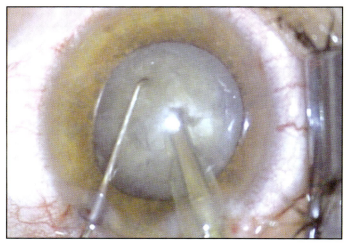

Fig. 10.25: Vertical chopping: the tip is sharp and need not be passed beyond the capsulorrhexis.

Phacoemulsification

8. With short bursts of power impale the phaco tip into the center of the nucleus.
9. With maximum vacuum hold the lens in position. The right hand holding the phaco handpiece should not be moved.
10. Score the lens with the chopper and bring it towards the phaco tip (Fig. 10.26).
11. Move the chopper laterally to split the nucleus (Fig. 10.27). Resist moving the phaco tip as the grip on the nucleus will be lost with the break in vacuum.
12. Repeat chopping to make smaller fragments.
13. Once a fragment has separated from the bulk of the nucleus, gradually build up the power to remove the nuclear material. Using higher power settings is counterproductive as it will repel the lens.

NB: When removing the last quadrant, protect the posterior capsule by decreasing vacuum and AFR, or by placing the second instrument behind the phaco tip.

Problems

1. Long operating time.
2. Difficult capsulorrhexis.
3. Because of poor visibility of the hydrodissection wave, too vigorous hydrodissection may result in posterior capsular blow-out.
4. Rotating and manipulating the nucleus may result zonular dehiscence because it occupies most of the lens.

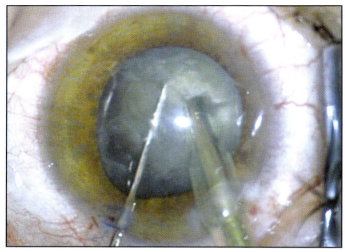

Fig. 10.26: Score the lens with the chopper (both vertical and horizontal chopping).

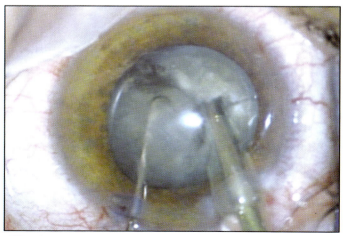

Fig. 10.27: Move the chopper laterally to complete the split.

5. Using very high power when sculpting may lead to a burn of the corneal wound.
6. Chopping may damage the anterior capsule and cause it to extend posteriorly resulting in a dropped nucleus.
7. Segmenting the nucleus may be difficult because the lower plates of the large nucleus may override.
8. Surge may occur as occlusion stops.
9. Increasing the power leads to repulsion of the nucleus.
10. Swirling hard small lens fragments may damage the corneal endothelium.

MANAGEMENT OF VITREOUS LOSS

Vitreous loss is a serious complication of phacoemulsification because it may compromise the visual outcome. A posterior capsular tear *per se* does not necessarily result in vitreous loss.

Vitreous Loss after Removal of All Nuclear Material

1. Plug the posterior capsular tear with Viscoat to prevent anterior vitreous herniation.
2. The vacuum and the cutting rate of the vitrector is controlled by the foot pedal. Less traction is exerted on the retina with a higher cut rate and lower vacuum but the procedure takes longer. Conversely,

a low cut rate with a high vacuum will result in swift removal of the vitreous gel but at a higher risk of traction on the retina.
3. Lower the height of the bottle containing irrigating fluid. This decreases turbulence in the anterior chamber, prevents enlargement of the tear and further loss of vitreous.
4. Insert the vitrector and the infusion cannula through the two sideports.
5. Clear *all* cortical remnants from the anterior a high cut rate chamber initially using and later high vacuum. Make small controlled movements of the cutter in the eye to minimize traction on the retina.
6. Remove all vitreous from the anterior chamber and a central bowl of the anterior vitreous.
7. Completed vitrectomy is characterized by free movement of the fluid in the anterior chamber and lack of movement of the iris while using the vitrector.
8. Inject viscoelastic between the iris and the anterior capsule and insert the IOL into the sulcus, between the anterior capsule and the iris.
9. Constrict the pupil by injecting Miochol.
10. With an iris repository sweep across the three incisions to ensure that they are free of vitreous.
11. Suture the corneal incision because it will not remain self-sealing.

Vitreous Loss before Removal of All Nuclear Material

1. A sudden deepening of the chamber and resistance to aspirating the nuclear fragments should alert the surgeon to a possibility of posterior capsular dehiscence.
2. Stop but do not remove instruments from the eye. Decompressing and recompressing the eye by frequent change of instruments encourages enlargement of the capsular tear and anterior vitreous prolapse.
3. Lower the bottle height to about 20 cm above the patient's eye.
4. Remove the second instrument from the eye but not the phaco.
5. Inject Viscoat underneath the nucleus to stabilize the nucleus and prevent anterior vitreous prolapse.
6. Remove the phaco from the eye.
7. Decide whether to continue with phaco or convert to an extracapsular cataract surgery depending on the amount of retained nuclear material and extent of the capsular tear.
8. Continuing phaco in an eye with a large capsular defect may result posterior dislocation of lens material unless a lens glide is inserted under the lens fragments. There is also a risk of retinal traction and endothelial damage.

9. If converting to extracapsular cataract surgery, enlarge the incision remembering that it has a triplanar configuration.

Impending or Actual Posterior Dislocation of Nuclear Fragments

Meticulously manage residual lens matter and vitreous and then refer to a vitreoretinal service as soon as possible.

Chapter 11

Irrigation and Aspiration

After completion of phacoemulsification, the cortical remnants are removed. Infusion is gravity dependent and is proportional to the height of the irrigation bottle. Aspiration is controlled with the automated system using the foot pedal or manually when using the Simcoe cannula. Bimanual I/A involves two separate cannulas. It provides good anterior chamber stability and facilitates removal of the sub-incisional cortex.

The technique is as follows:

1. Insert the I/A cannulas downwards through the two sideports. Difficulty may be due to a soft eye; make the eye firm by injecting BSS through the main corneal incision.
2. Place the cannula underneath the anterior capsule with the aspiration port facing upwards.
3. Press the foot pedal to create a vacuum to grip the anterior cortical lens matter (Fig. 11.1).
4. Use vacuum to hold and bring the cortical material to the center (Fig. 11.2).
5. Increase the vacuum to aspirate lens matter (Fig. 11.3).
6. Repeat the procedure till all the soft lens matter is aspirated.
7. Small nuclear fragments or harder cortical material can be crushed between the tips of the I/A cannula.

IRRIGATION AND ASPIRATION

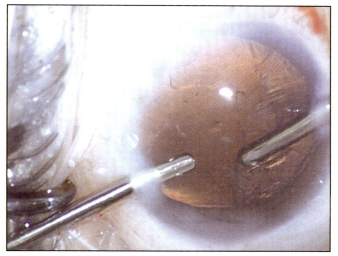

Fig. 11.1: Gripping of cortical lens matter using vacuum.

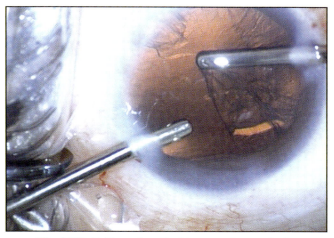

Fig. 11.2: Pulling of cortical lens matter centrally.

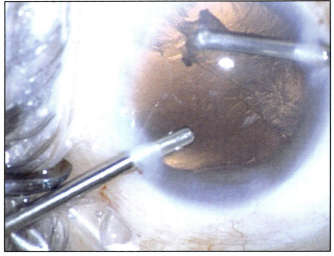

Fig. 11.3: Aspiration of cortical lens matter.

Chapter 12

Insertion of IOL and Completion

The following technique describes implantation of an injectable IOL.

1. Fill the capsular bag and the anterior chamber with Healon to push the posterior capsule backwards, open the capsular bag and iron out capsular folds (Fig. 12.1). This facilitates insertion of IOL into the capsular bag and reduces the risk of posterior capsular tear.

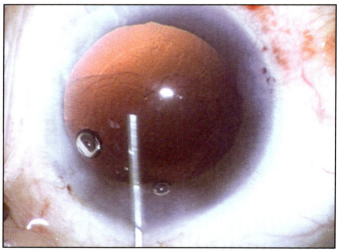

Fig. 12.1: Injection of viscoelastic.

2. Stabilize the eye and enlarge the main incision to approximately 3.2 mm.
3. Rotate the keratome laterally to make the internal opening should be slightly wider than the outer (Fig. 12.2).

INSERTION OF IOL AND COMPLETION

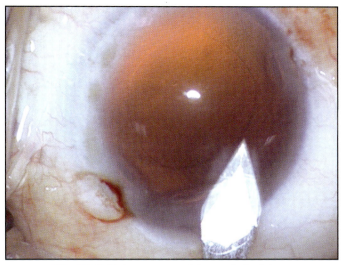

Fig. 12.2: Enlargement of the main incision.

4. Take the IOL out of its packaging and place on a flat surface. A small amount of Healon can be placed underneath the IOL for stability.
5. Two forceps are used to fold the IOL. Grooved forceps hold the IOL and the other hold the folded IOL for implantation (Fig. 12.3).
6. Place the grooved forceps at the junction of the haptic and the optic of the IOL (Fig. 12.3).
7. Gradually increase the force as the IOL starts folding.
8. Use the other forceps to hold the folded over lens (Fig. 12.4).

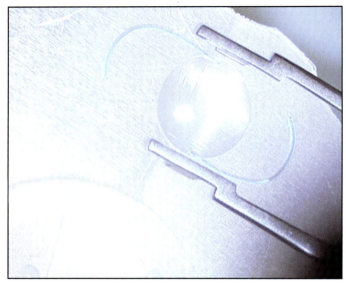

Fig. 12.3: Folding the IOL.

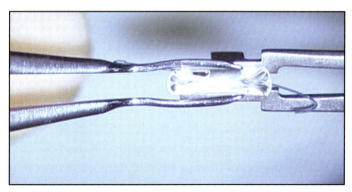

Fig. 12.4: Holding the IOL.

Insertion of IOL and Completion

9. Place the metal parallel and touching the metal of the grooved forceps ensuring that the tips do not protrude beyond the IOL.
10. Ensure that the haptics are not caught between the forceps.
11. Insert the leading haptic into the eye (Fig. 12.5).
12. Place the folded IOL close to the main incision and press down on the posterior lip of the incision.
13. Gently advance the IOL. Watch the leading haptic and manipulate the lens so that it enters the capsular bag (Fig. 12.6).

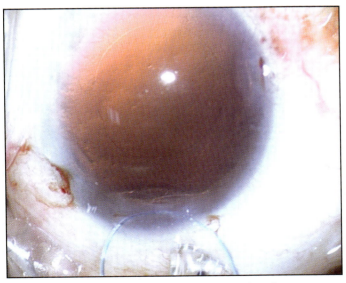

Fig. 12.5: Insertion of the leading haptic.

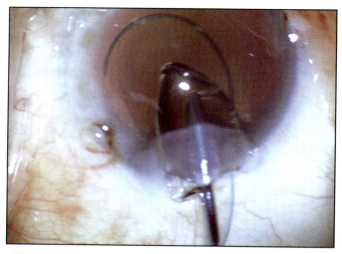

Fig. 12.6: Insertion of the optic: aim downwards so that the leading haptic goes underneath the anterior capsule.

14. Rotate the forceps so that the fold of the IOL lies anteriorly and release (Fig. 12.7).
15. As the IOL gently unfolds insert the dialler in the groove between the haptic and optic. This gives maximum mechanical advantage to rotating the lens inside the capsular bag (Fig. 12.8).
16. When the IOL is inserted into the bag it should be centred with the dialler (Fig. 12.9).
17. Aspirate residual viscoelastic.
18. Seal the sideports with a jet of BSS but the main incision need not be sealed (Fig. 12.10).

INSERTION OF IOL AND COMPLETION 127

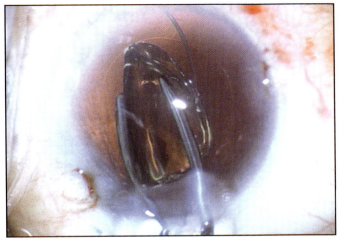

Fig. 12.7: Unfolding of the IOL.

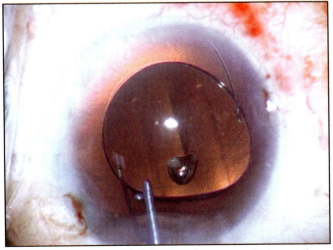

Fig. 12.8: Insertion of dialler into the groove between the haptic and optic.

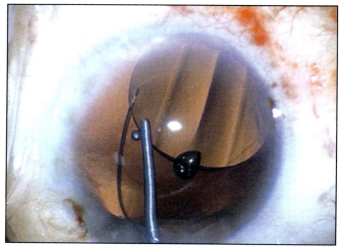

Fig. 12.9: Dialling of IOL.

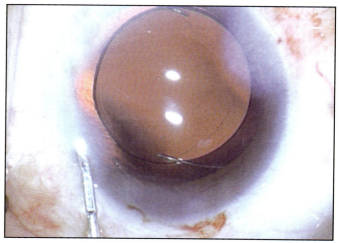

Fig. 12.10: Hydration of sideports.

INSERTION OF IOL AND COMPLETION

19. Check the integrity of the incisions by pressing on the surface of the cornea to increase intraocular pressure. Leakage is detected with a dry cellulose sponge held at the main incision and sideports.
20. Give a subconjunctival injection of antibiotic and steroid.
21. Remove the speculum.

NB: Drape removal is often the most painful part of the operation; use a wet gauze to gently peel the drape.

Index

A

Adjustment of filters 39
Advantage of phacoemulsification 56
Akinesia 22
Anaesthesia 21
  general 31
  infiltrative 23
  sub-Tenon 24
  topical 22
    advantages 22
    disadvantages 23
Anaesthetic agents
  amethocaine 22
  benoxinate 22
  lignocaine gel 22
  proxymetacaine 22
Analgesia 22
Anterior capsular tear 101
Aspiration 117
Aspiration bypass system (ABS) 52
Aspiration flow rate 45
Associated ocular disease 17
  glaucoma
    filtration bleb 18
    intraocular pressure 18
  previous vitrectomy
    lack of vitreous support 19
    other factors 20
    uncertain visual outcome 19
  pseudoexfoliation 20
  uveitis
    control of 17
    identification of potential limitations 17

B

Bowl formation 106

C

Capsular flap 75
Capsular tear 122
Capsulorrhexis 11, 71
  principles 72
  special situations
    difficult visualization of the anterior capsule 77
    rhexis running out 78
    weak zonules 78
  start of capsulorrhexis 74
  technique 72
Cavitation 53
Cavitation bubble 53
Centripetal vector force 72
Cohesivity 68
Completed vitrectomy 114
Conjunctival sac 35

Corneal distortion 96

D

Diabetic retinopathy 4
Diaphragmatic pump 50
Divide and conquer technique 90
Draping 36

E

Elasticity 68
Emulsification 53
Endothelial dystrophy 12
Endothelial trauma 102
Epinuclear cushion 99
Examination 5
    anterior chamber depth
        shallow 13
        very deep 13
    cornea 11
    external features 7
        chronic dacryocystitis 10
        deep set eyes and small palpebral fissures 7
        hearing aids 8
        infected contralateral socket 10
        staphylococcal blepharitis 8
    grading of nucleus
        grade 1 5
        grade 2 5
        grade 3 6
        grade 4 7
        grade 5 7
    pupil size 11

F

Flow pumps 50
Folded IOL 123

G

Globe perforation 31
Grade 3 nucleus 90
    removal of lens quadrants (Conquer) 97
        problems 101
        technique 97
    sculpting (Divide) 90
        problems 94
        technique 90

H

Hard nucleus 106
    problems 111
    technique 106
Height of irrigating bottle 44
Horizontal chopping 110, 112
Hydration of sideports 128
Hydrodissection 81
    problems
        inadequate hydrodissection 84
        vigorous hydrodissection 85
    purpose 82
    technique 82
Hydrodissection fluid wave 83

I

Incision
    location 60
        clear corneal incision 60
        limbal incision 60
        on-axis phaco incision 63
        sclerocorneal incision 62
        superior incision 63
        superotemporal incision 63
        temporal incision 62
    shape 63

three-plane incision 63
three-plane self-sealing incision 64
Infusion 118
Injection of viscoelastic 122
Insertion of IOL and completion 121
  technique 122
Iodine 35
Iris 100
Iris trauma 97
Irrigating bottle 44
Irrigation 117

J

Jackhammer pneumatic drill effect 53

K

Kelman tip 51
Keratome 122

M

Management of vitreous loss 113
  impending or actual posterior dislocation of nuclear fragments 116
  vitreous loss after removal of all nuclear material 113
  vitreous loss before removal of all nuclear material 115
Medical history
  diabetes 3
    diabetic retinopathy 3
    other problems 3
  other considerations
    anticoagulants 4
    hypertension 4

O

Ocular history 2
  refraction
    high myopia 3
    hypermetropia 3
  trauma
    blunt trauma 2
    penetrating trauma 2

P

Paracentesis 56
  advantages of two sideports 57
  purposes 56
  technique 56
Peribulbar haemorrhage 31
Peribulbar injection 28
  problems 31
  technique 28
Peristaltic machines 45
Peristaltic pump 50
Phaco 91
Phacodynamics 43
Phacoemulsification 53, 89, 118
  aim 90
Phacoemulsifiers 49
  designs 50
  handpiece 50
  phaco tip 50
    diameter 52
    distal bevel 52
    other modifications 52
    shape 50
    sleeve 52
Posterior capsular tear 101
Preparation for surgery 33
  communication 41
  foot pedal 40
  microscope settings 37
  position of the table and head 34

preparation of the eye 35
Pseudoplasticity 68

R

Rhexis 72
Ripping 72
Rotary vane pump 50

S

Scroll pump 50
See-saw 94
Shearing 72
Simcoe cannula 56
Soft nucleus 102
    problems 103
    technique 102
Soft shell 70
Soft shell technique 108
Sub-Tenon injection 24
    problems 25
    technique 25
Surface adhesion (coatability) 68
Surge 46

T

Tenon capsule 26
Transmission of acoustic waves 53
Trench formation 93

U

Uveitis-glaucoma-hyphema syndrome 72

V

Vacuum 45
Vacuum pumps 50
Venturi pump 50
Vertical chopping 110
Viscoelastics 67,68
    clinical uses
        if capsulorrhexis is running out to the periphery 69
        improving visibility 69
        in small posterior capsular tears 69
        in small pupils 69
        soft shell technique 69
    properties
        cohesive viscoelastic 68
        dispersive viscoelastics 69
Viscosity 68

W

Warfarin 4

Z

Zonular weakness 96